Table of Contents

"Buy This Diet Book First"

This Book Will Identify The Key You Need To Know To Succeed In Losing Weight

There are over 50,000 diet and weight loss books out there based on recent research. Many people buy multiple books, in a seemingly never ending quest to find the "answer" for them. But those books do not address the main issue driving weight loss success.

This book will identifies for you what that main weight loss program issue is, and how to solve it for you, individually.

This books boils down the key facts and learned experiences for you all in just one easy to read book.

This book is probably the one single book will get you need. So read this book before buying other books, checking out the latest weight loss fads, joining and paying for weight loss programs. You will achieve results you want earlier, and save yourself a lot of frustration, time and money.

The Key To A Successful Weight Loss Program

No matter how many ways you look at weight loss, the bottom line is that you either gain weight or lose weight based on one factor. That factor is your net calories taken in less calories expended. If you take in more calories than you expend, you gain weight. If you expend more calories than you take in, you lose weight. Period.

So, it stands to reason that if you want to lose weight, you need to take in less calories than you expend. The concept is simple, but yet it is very important to establish this as the foundation for moving forward to a successful weight loss plan.

If you can increase the calories you expend, that will help you lose weight, but experience shows that most people do not reliably increase their calories expended on a consistent basis. And, the amount of effort to burn the calories required to offset overeating can quickly become impractical. Example; it takes about 1 hour of exercise to burn off the calories in just two slices of bread.

Therefore, realistically, the most effective way you will lose weight is to **reduce the calories you take into your body** every day. This is a FACT.

Now that we have established **"what"** to do (eat less calories), the next step is **"how"** to do it.

How to Make a Diet Plan Happen For You

As stated, we know "what" we need to do (take in less calories than we expend each day), so we turn our attention to "how" to do it. **How is the key!**

This book focuses on helping you with the "how" of getting a diet successfully into practice and working.

Reality Check; Eyes Wide Open And What Lies Ahead

Most of the books, programs, clubs, fads, are really trying to address the issue of "how" to lose weight. But, they do not talk to the primary problem most people have with successful dieting. They talk to types of foods, different food groups to eat, or avoid, healthy foods, junk foods, times to eat, portions to eat, how to cook, blenders to buy, times and frequency to eat, etc. Many try to make dieting seem like "fun". These books also can make weight loss all seem to be so easy. They portray smiling, happy, slim people, who seem so darn happy. This portrayal may help sell books, but it is misleading and creates a false perception, as real weight loss requires some level of hard work and commitment. The dieting we know is hard work, not our first idea of being" fun", and involves doing less of something we like to do, eat !

So the first thing we need to do is sign up for the realization that dieting will not be "fun".

Honest Self- Assessment

While there is no doubt that certain foods are healthier than others, and certain foods are more calories and would counterproductive to losing weight, these diets do not address the primary issue that people have in successfully losing weight. This primary issue is either a person **HAS** the self-discipline to control and manage the food and drink they eat or, try as they might, the person **DOES NOT HAVE** that level of self- discipline and control, so they end up eating more than they know they should and do not lose weight.

In theory, every person has the ability to manage what they eat.

No one is forcing anyone to eat. Eating is the conscious action of the individual. There are many examples where dieters have lost weight if they want it enough. This means wanting the results more than the temptation and satisfaction from eating. TV Shows like Biggest Loser show such examples. No one is saying it is easy or fun, but it IS possible, and you can do it too!

The people who are successful seem to get a clear understanding as to "why" they want to lose weight, and that "why" is a meaningful reason for them.

If the reason is not legitimate for them, it is likely that the temptation and gratification they get from eating will overtake them.

The successful people get themselves to a point where they make a commitment, understand the work and trials that will be involved, and consciously say" I CAN do this".

So prospective candidates for weight loss can be categorized into the following groups:

1. Can individually manage what they eat,
2. Need assistance to manage what they eat,
3. Will not truly commit to any diet plan.

If you are lucky enough to be a person in Group #1 you individually can muster the self-control and discipline to limit what you eat, and expend more calories than you take in, then you do not need to read this book or any diet plan any further. You can lose weight and diet on your own, without additional assistance. Congratulations!

And, if you are person in Group #3, the truth is that unless you have some level of true commitment, realizing the hard work and self-control required, <u>no plan or program will work</u>. A person may have temporary weight losses, but will later regain the weight, and may yo-yo up and down.

Without some true commitment, unless the person is in a locked room and fed only by a guard, the person would find a way to cheat, sneak food, make excuses, break the weight loss plan and gain weight.

From a reality perspective, the following maybe a harsh "tough-love" statement, but if you are in Group #3, please recognize that in order to be successful, you need to transition your mind set and commitment up to be at least in Group #2.

Finally, this leaves us with the people in Group #2. This is probably the largest group, by far. We all wish we were in Group #1, but, as difficult as it may be to admit, we need to be honest and look at the facts. Many people do NOT have the self-discipline and will power to control the calorie level of what they consume. They need some form of help and assistance. If you are in Group #2, know that you are not alone, far from it. Eating habits are very, very difficult to break, and restricting calorie intake in our "food everywhere, available all the time" society requires a level of commitment.

There should be no shame in accepting that help is needed. People have evolved through times when food was scarce, so eating as much as available was an advantage for survival. Many bright people are overweight, so it is not a matter of intelligence.

Some people find a level of comfort or control in eating. These urges are tough to overcome or redirect. Eating is also pleasurable, so limiting it means a reduction in pleasurable and gratifying experiences. Dieting is tough. It's OK, you are not alone.

But it is important to recognize and accept if you are in Group #2, you need help if you truly want to lose weight. If you are buying diet books, you probably can count yourself as one who is looking for and needs assistance. If you have tried to lose weight in the past without success, then it stands to reason you probably need assistance. Be honest with yourself. Your chances for successful dieting depends your honest assessment with yourself.

The Bottom Line is "How"

The bottom line is that the key success factor in losing weight is not the diet plan itself but **how** you will stay true to the plan you choose successfully.

Consider an absurd hypothetical case, just to make a point. Picture yourself stranded on a desert island, with hardly any food resources. To survive you had to ration the little food available, just to stay alive. In this extreme case, anyone would obviously lose weight.

The point again being that we are overweight because we are not on a desert island, food is over abundant and available, and do not have the will power to restrict our calorie intake such that we maintain a healthy BMI.

Once you realize and accept that you need help and assistance to make a successful diet happen for you, **the next step is to look at the types of help and assistance available.**

After you make the commitment, you need to determine which assistance works for you. Usually it is NOT a book or gimmick, but how you can best avoid eating.

Types of Help and Assistance Available

As mentioned, there are all kinds of books, fads, programs, etc. out there to be "helpful", but the ultimate effectiveness of all of these boil down to if they help you overcome a less than complete 100% level of self-control and discipline.

The more remote and far away the help is, the less likely influence they have. The less influence the weight loss program has, the more self-control and commitment is required from the individual. So called "fat farms" and in-residence weight loss programs have a lot of influence, as these are hands programs with 24/7 personal, individual attention. The next level down are programs where you pay, then go in to meetings and get weighed in front of people, or get food portions delivered to your home. These have some level of third party group influence. Another level down from that is to work with a non-paid, partner, typically someone you know and are close to, to help manage your weight loss plan. The partner can be a spouse, roommate, etc. that acts as your trainer, helper, coordinator. Finally, books, apps and diet plans alone have the least involvement of others, so are the least level of direct influence.

None of the above solution is better or worse than the other, per se, it just depends on what will be effective for the individual.

Where you assess your level of commitment and ability to stand firm, with strong will power in the face of temptation and match that to the level of weight loss program assistance is up to you.

Remember, most people cannot do it alone. If you are in this category, do not be afraid to enlist help. If you are hesitant, this will hold you back.

But, weight loss is an extremely private matter. Most people do not want to let others know they are trying to diet. Dieters already feel a bit sheepish about the fact they are overweight already, so letting others know is one of the last things they want to do.

In the following sections, we will address the types of help available, and an option that can work for many Group #2 dieters.

The Assistance Plan That CAN Work For YOU

So, unless you can afford the time and expense to check yourself in to a residence program, you need the next best thing for assistance in your efforts to help you manage your weight.

You have tried weight loss programs, but always seem to eat more than you should or stray from the plan. So this book suggests you get that extra boost of help from another person who will help you.

A very effective way to control your calorie intake is to enlist the help of another person to assist in managing what you eat. This is a non-paid helper who you know and trust. We will call them your Personal Weight Loss Assistant (PWLA).

 It is best if this person lives in the same household with you. It can be a spouse, a roommate, a brother, sister and even a teenage child.

The PWLA will relive you of the stress, anxiety and guilt of giving in to weaknesses. You will feel comforted that you have help and compassion to ward off impulses and temptations.

You can work out a day by day diet plan, and agree on it ahead of time. So, the PWLA is YOUR assistant, so you make the decisions. The effectiveness comes in two key areas:

1. Though you are making the decisions, your PWLA will see what you are deciding, so this alone will help keep you true to a sensible weight loss diet plan,
2. You will empower your PWLA to help you most I your times of strongest temptation, when you are wavering and perhaps about to fall off the diet. The PWLA will help you by being an extra step to help keep you on your diet and help you from inappropriate eating. More about this later.

So what we are saying here is that most dieters know what to do, but the problem comes in when they have to try to stay on the diet all by themselves, and need assistance. If you have another person who will help you in this way, and if you can willingly accept the other person as authorized to manage your eating, it will help <u>you</u> achieve <u>your</u> weight loss goals.

Working Together With Your Personal Weight Loss Assistant

To help facilitate this arrangement, it is important to be very clear as to roles and responsibilities. To help facilitate this understanding, it may be helpful to review, agree to and even sign the below draft Assistance Agreement. You can change it to what best works for your situation.

You know without any doubt that **it is possible** to eat less. The obstacle is a lack of will power and discipline, which is so common and understandable. You need to try to create an environment where you get help with the discipline. Of course, even with any type of help, if a person is not truly committed, they can sabotage the plan, cheat, sneak food, and undermine the process. So, some level of cooperation and commitment is required. If you can do this, you will achieve success. The PWLA is your assistant, not a drill sergeant or lion trainer.

The main thing is to prepare in advance of how you will act when temptation comes, and how do you want the PWLA to act. It is NOT fair to the PWLA to have to stand up to ridicule, yelling, begging or other behaviors that will make them feel bad.

In olden times, when a soldier was wounded on the battlefield need to have some sort of surgery or a bullet removed, without anesthesia, they would have either a few strong men hold the soldier down, or one woman. The point is that if the patient fights with all their might to get out of the situation, a lot of force is needed, whereas if the patient is willing to cooperate, force is not needed, just some assistance.

The PWLA fills this role. The PWLA is the aide of the dieter, not a force to resist and fight against.

The dieter needs to treat the PWLA with respect and as a person who is trying to help and assist the dieter.

If you do not have anyone handy who will work with you, you will need to get the support you need elsewhere. Programs and clubs can work but are more remote, and they are very expensive.

Assistance Agreement (template)

This Agreement is created by _____,
(Dieter), who assigns to _____,
Dieter's Personal Weight Loss Assistant (PWLA)
approval responsibility for all calorie intake of eating
and drinking by Dieter, beginning on
date_____ and ending on date
_____.

Dieter understands this request of Dieter's PWLA is
one to help the Dieter, and Dieter agrees it is a kind
and helpful act for the Dieter's PWLA to enter this
contract.

Dieter and Dieter's PWLA should agree each week, in
advance, in writing, of the upcoming week's diet plan
(Plan), meal by meal, with daily calorie totals. (Diet
Plans should be healthy, nutritious, and provide the
nourishment requirements of Dieter, to be approved
by a Physician as appropriate)

During the week, Dieter agrees to only eat and drink
what is in the weeks Plan or what the Dieter's PWLA
agrees is appropriate towards the Dieter's goal of
losing weight.

If and when the Dieter is tempted to stray from the
agreed upon diet Plan, Dieter directs Dieter's PWLA
to politely, but firmly help Dieter resist temptation
and not give in.

Dieter agrees not to cheat. If the Dieter cheats, the Agreement immediately ends. The PWLA cannot be asked to be party to an agreement where the Dieter is not cooperating. And PWLA is expressly not responsible for 24/7 surveillance of the Dieter.

Dieter will not have any foods, snacks, sweets, etc. not on the agreed to weekly diet Plan in the household or accessible for snacking.

Dieter will weigh themselves once a week and Dieter's PWLA will write down the results and keep track of them.

Optional: If Dieter breaks from the Plan, or puts pressure on the Dieter's PWLA, Dieter agrees to do the following favor for Dieter's PWLA_____ (example: do a task for the PWLA).

Date: _____

Signed below

_____

Dieter

_____

Dieter's PWLA

Tips to Help You Lose Weight and Stay on Your Diet Plan

The below "tips" can be helpful in a weight loss program. You do not have to use or follow all of them. Use the ones that you feel will work for you.

First, know and believe that you CAN succeed. Know that you must make a serious, conscious commitment to improve your chance for success. Know and accept you are making commitment to endure some discomfort when the urge to eat or cheat come along. If you are half- heartedly starting out, you may be susceptible to lose control when the going gets tough.

You must find the thing that works for you as to your "why", in order to stay on track and not give in, when the temptation to eat comes along. Plan ahead and envision that time of temptation coming, and act out what you will do. Then, when the time actually does come, follow the actions you have prepared.

When temptation comes, it can also help to try to distract yourself, do something else, delay, redirect your thoughts, or make it a point not to give in. Think about what is the thing that will help you not succumb to temptation to eat comes along. The longer you can delay the better. Each day and week, the delay period can be longer and longer, until you break the urge and habit.

Some research shows that you **can break a habit if you can avoid doing it for 22 days**. After that, the mind and body have passed a major milestone and been retrained so that the habit is broken.

Try to stay away from the foods and drinks that are your weaknesses. If you do not have these things in the household, you will be less tempted and less likely to slip up and go off your Plan.

If you cannot control yourself at the grocery store, have someone else shop for you.

If you have kids and some of your weakness items are for them, you must either still not have those items around, or have them in a separate area, out of sight.

Try to reduce the amounts of times you eat out at restaurants, eat fast food, or carryout.

Slowly drink a glass of water before meals. Slowly drink a glass of water before eating anything.

You can eat more volume of lower calorie foods that high calorie foods.

Try to limit high calorie foods, like starchy foods, sugars, breads and alcohol.

Slow down when you eat. Chew 33 times before you swallow. Try to drag out the time it takes to eat as much as possible.

If you have a weak time, set up another activity to take your mind off food at these times. Preoccupy yourself somehow.

If you have to eat outside of the plan, try to eat carrots or vegetables that contain a very little amount of calories.

If you have to have something besides vegetables, try to snack on Cheerios. Eat them one at a time. Take as long as you can with each one, so as much time as possible passes.

Try to visualize, in as much detail as possible, what motivates you most for your goal. Whether that is a better looking body, or better shape and flexibility, or healthier feeling.

Envision yourself how you want to look and how much better you will feel.

Envision that the urges to eat are personified by someone or something you very strongly dislike. Imagine that they are trying to control you and force you to eat. When you do eat, they laugh and enjoy it.

Try to get to the point of feeling some level of hunger, as a good thing. Congratulate yourself and know you are making progress when this happens.

Congratulate yourself for EVERY small victory and step. Progress starts slowly and in small steps. These are the most difficult.

Try to set up things you must do first before you eat anything. This will take up time, and take away some of the anticipation of pleasure from eating. It should be something you do not like to do. Examples: Do 10 pushups, do 20 sit ups, spend 15 minutes cleaning or doing household chores, walk around the block, or take a taste of something you do not like the taste of.

Put a bell on your refrigerator and pantry doors.

Put a mirror on the refrigerator at eye level, and a scale in front of the refrigerator. Put a bell on the door. Look at the mirror and get on the scale every time you approach.

When tempted, delay, delay, delay. Delay becomes not eating, over time.

Conclusion

To sum up,

- You really already know "what" you need to do (restrict caloric intake), so you do not need more information on this aspect

- "How" to do it and stay with it, is the main question

- The answer for you depends on you. Assess your level of will power and commitment

- Select the level of influence and assistance that matches your need based on your level of will power and commitment. This is the key. The right level of help with the dieter's individual ability to stay on a plan.

- The PWLA option is a level and form of assistance that will fit the needs of most dieters. More assistance than going it alone, or but less than in residence programs, PWLA provides just the right level of boost to the dieter when they need I most. PWLA helps with temporary lapses in will power to keep the dieter on plan. PWLA has the added benefit of being no cost.

You CAN do it, if you want it enough!!

IMPORTANT NOTES FOR ALL READERS

IMPORTANT: The above is practical advice suitable for most people, but in all cases, the reader should consult their physician in matters of diet and weight loss.

IMPORTANT: To determine your healthy weight level many use the Body Mass Index number (BMI).

IMPORTANT: Many prefer people do not uses chemicals, diet pills or substances to lose weight as a first resort, as there can be side-effects, etc.

Dedications

First, this book is dedicated to my wife, Elizabeth, who has supported me in my efforts to write this book.

Second, to all those out there who make the effort to manage their weight and who maintain a positive commitment achieving their goals.

Success to all!

J. F. Sebastian

www.ingramcontent.com/pod-product-compliance
Lightning Source LLC
Chambersburg PA
CBHW072015280526
45788CB00005B/2060

* 9 7 8 1 5 3 0 7 8 6 3 9 8 *